Living with heart failure – a guide for patients

Professor Martin R Cowie

*National Heart & Lung Institute,
Imperial College, and
Royal Brompton Hospital, London*

BLADON
MEDICAL
PUBLISHING

© 2003
by Bladon Medical Publishing

12 New Street, Chipping Norton, Oxfordshire OX7 5LJ, UK

First published 2003

All rights reserved. No part of this publication may be reproduced, stored in a retrieval system, or transmitted in any form or by any means, electronic, mechanical, photocopying, recording or otherwise without the prior permission of the copyright owner.

The Authors have asserted their right under the Copyright, Designs and Patents Act, 1988, to be identified as the Authors of this work.

Always refer to the manufacturer's Prescribing Information before prescribing drugs cited in this book.

British Library Cataloguing in Publication Data.

A catalogue record for this title is available from the British Library

ISBN 1-904218-22-9

Professor Martin R Cowie. Living with heart failure – a guide for patients

Design and production:
Design Online Limited, 21 Cave Street, Oxford

Printed by
Talleres Gráficos Hostench, s.a.,
Venezuela, 87–93, 08019 Barcelona, Spain

Distributed by
Plymbridge Distributors Ltd, Estover Road, Plymouth
PL6 7PY, UK

Contents

Chapter 1
Introduction: Heart failure is not the end of the road … 1

Chapter 2
How should my heart work? … 5

Chapter 3
So why did it go wrong? … 11

Chapter 4
How will the doctor decide I have heart failure? … 17

Chapter 5
How is heart failure treated? … 27

Chapter 6
How will treatment affect my everyday life? … 41

Appendix
Sources of help and information … 51

Index … 55

Chapter 1

Introduction: Heart failure is not the end of the road

So you've been told you have heart failure. The first thing that you need to know about your illness is that, whatever the name implies, heart failure doesn't mean that your heart has given up or is about to stop working. Rather, it means that your heart is weakened and is having difficulty in pumping as hard as it would like to do to keep up with your body's need for oxygen and other nutrients, particularly when you are doing any exercise.

Heart failure may range in severity from mild to severe. Depending on the severity of your illness, you may experience some or all of the following symptoms at some point:

- Shortness of breath either when sitting or more usually during physical activity or at night when lying in bed
- Tiredness
- Swollen ankles and feet, and maybe also swelling of the legs, groin and abdomen
- Dry cough
- Loss of appetite, constipation or abdominal bloating

These are symptoms that are likely to have a tremendous impact on your ability to do the everyday things that previously you took for granted, such as shopping, housework and running for the bus. Some people find that their symptoms make them less and less active, perhaps forcing them to give up work and even their hobbies. Modern treatment for heart failure can greatly improve your symptoms and allow you to return to many, if not all, of these activities.

In the UK, doctors identify about 65,000 new cases of heart failure each year. At any one time there are at least 750,000 people in the UK with heart failure – roughly 1–2% of the population.

If you assume that your GP has about 2000 people on his or her practice list, that means that, as well as you, there may be another 20 people with heart failure in your area. By medical standards this makes heart failure a very common illness, roughly as common as diabetes.

Introduction: Heart failure is not the end of the road

Although in most cases, there is no cure for heart failure, it doesn't mean that you've reached the end of the road. It's not a death sentence. In fact, just like diabetes it is an illness that many people are able to live with for many years. By taking the right medicines and making a few simple adjustments to your lifestyle, you will probably find that you are able to control your symptoms very well.

Reading this book will help you to understand more about your heart failure, the treatment you are likely to be given by your doctor and the important part that you and your family can play in helping to manage your own illness and its impact upon your life.

Chapter 2

How should my heart work?

In order to help you learn more about heart failure and how to reduce its effect on your life, you need to understand a little about what the heart does and how it should work.

The blood circulation

For your body to keep working properly, all the tissues and organs within it need a constant supply of oxygen and other nutrients such as the proteins, sugars, fats and vitamins that you provide it with at each mealtime. The tissues themselves get their supplies of these nutrients from the blood, which flows around the body within a closed network of blood vessels, just as water flows through a central heating system.

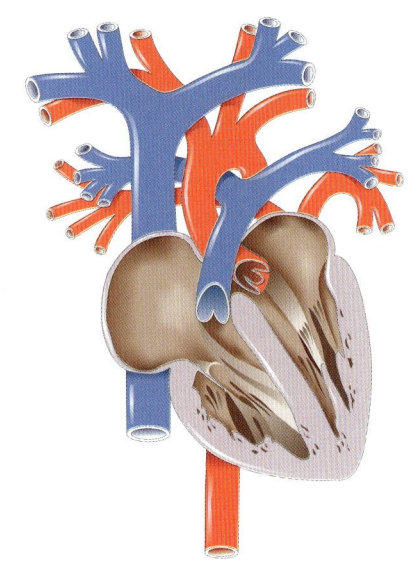

But whereas a central heating system has a boiler to keep pumping hot water around the system, a pump made of muscle, called the heart, drives the circulatory system within your body.

The heart is made up of four hollow chambers. The two upper chambers, the atria, are connected to two powerful pumping lower chambers, the ventricles, by means of valves designed to keep the blood flowing in the right direction. The ventricles are, in turn, connected to the main arteries to the lungs and the rest of the body by two other valves, which keep the blood flowing in the right direction.

This four-chambered arrangement allows the heart to keep blood circulating around your body continuously in a single direction, picking up oxygen and nutrients and delivering them to all your tissues and organs.

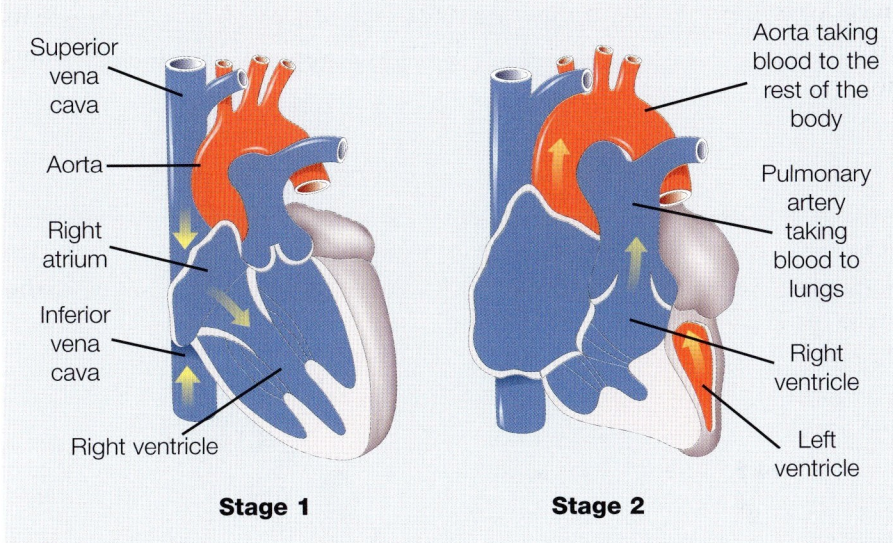

Figure 2.1. *Stage 1* – Used blood (from the body) is pumped into the right ventricle by the right atrium. Simultaneously oxygenated blood (from the lungs) is pumped into the left ventricle by the left atrium (not shown). *Stage 2* – The used blood in the right ventricle is pumped to the lungs (via the pulmonary artery) and, at the same time, oxygenated blood in the left ventricle is pumped to the rest of the body (via the aorta) (not shown).

How the circulation works

The right side of the heart pumps blood through the pulmonary artery to the lungs. Here it picks up oxygen from the air that we inhale each time we breathe. This oxygen-carrying blood is then returned to the left side of the heart through the pulmonary veins, and is then pumped out to the rest of the body through the aorta, the body's main artery.

After blood has been circulated to all the tissues through ever-smaller blood vessels (the smallest are called capillaries) most of the oxygen and nutrients have been removed. The blood then returns towards the heart through ever-larger blood vessels called veins. All the veins of the body come together before entering the heart to form the superior and inferior vena cava, which connect to the right side of the heart.

From the right side of the heart, this 'deoxygenated' blood is again pumped to the lungs to pick up more oxygen.

How does the heat beat?

The body needs a great deal of oxygen – in a normal adult, the heart beats about 70 times every minute and pumps about 5 litres of blood through the body's circulatory system. The amount of blood that is pumped by the heart depends on the amount of activity that you are doing – when you are physically active, the body needs more oxygen and nutrients, and so the heart pumps faster and pumps more blood with each beat. When you are resting, the heart pumps more slowly.

During each heart beat, the chambers of the heart first relax (a phase called diastole) and fill up with blood before they contract and expel blood out into the circulation (a phase called systole). The two atria relax and contract together, as do the two ventricles.

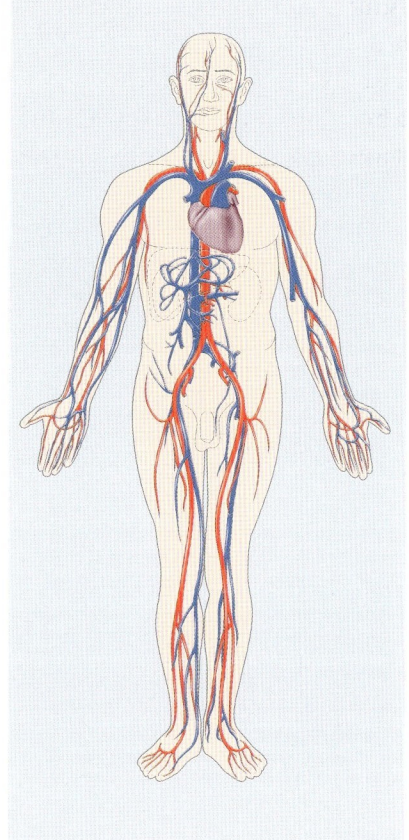

Figure 2.2. The circulatory system – blood is pumped out from the heart through the arteries and returns to the heart through the veins.

The heart has a natural 'pacemaker' which ensures it keeps beating throughout life. This pacemaker is found in the wall of the right atrium, and the electrical impulses that make the heart beat spread out from here through the whole heart in a carefully controlled way. The body can speed up the pacemaker (and thus speed up the heart beat) in response to the body's needs such as exercise or stress.

Using a stethoscope a doctor can listen to the sounds the heart makes through the pumping cycle. Problems with the heart valves and the heart muscle can often be picked up in this way, although other tests often need to be done to provide further information. The rumbling sound made by blood rushing through a damaged valve is called a 'murmur.'

Chapter 3

So why did it go wrong?

Our hearts have to do a lot of work to get us through life. Even if you have had a relatively inactive life, by the time you reach the age of 65 your heart will have beaten around 2,500,000,000 times.

That represents a lot of work, so maybe it's not surprising that as we get older our hearts may start to work less well; with time, most people's hearts lose some degree of pumping efficiency. In patients with heart failure, this is serious enough to result in symptoms such as breathlessness and swollen ankles. In general, most people are over 70 years of age when they are diagnosed with heart failure.

Any condition that forces the heart to work harder than it needs to over a period of years can increase the chance of it weakening and of heart failure developing. For some people, damage to the heart can occur more suddenly, such as after a large heart attack.

Doctors believe that heart failure is becoming more common. This is partly because we are all living longer nowadays, but also because doctors have being getting steadily better at treating other problems such as heart attacks so that more people survive a heart attack but may have a damaged heart which may start failing months to years after the heart attack.

Heart failure can affect both men and women, but men are at a higher risk of heart failure at all ages – chiefly because coronary heart disease (angina and heart attack) is more common in men. However, because women on average live longer than men, in older age groups the numbers are more finely balanced. In addition, there is some evidence to suggest that black people are more likely to develop heart failure, particularly due to high blood pressure, than white people. People of South Asian origin may be at a higher risk of heart failure due to a higher risk of diabetes and coronary heart disease. However, it is important to remember that heart failure can affect both men and women of any age and of any ethnic origin.

How the body copes with a failing heart

Even though your heart muscle may get progressively weaker and lose its pumping efficiency, your body still demands a constant supply of oxygen and nutrients. In order to maintain these supplies, your body triggers several mechanisms that try to ensure the heart keeps working as hard as it can.

As a short-term measure, it sets off an emergency response by releasing hormones, such as adrenaline and noradrenaline from the adrenal glands and nerve endings. These increase your heart rate and make the heart pump harder to increase the amount of blood it pumps out to the body. Although this has a benefit to the body, in a patient with long-term heart failure it can actually cause the heart to deteriorate further.

Another compensatory mechanism involves the kidneys reducing the amount of salt (or sodium) and water that they excrete in the urine. This leads to retention of fluid, which increases the volume of blood in the circulation. Having a higher volume of fluid causes the heart muscle to stretch and to contract more forcefully, increasing the pumping ability of the heart. But as heart failure progresses, some of this excess fluid can escape from the circulation, and accumulate in different parts of your body. This is why you get swelling (or oedema) particularly in the legs and feet. If the fluid begins to collect in your lungs, it can lead to shortness of breath, causing breathing problems, especially when you lie down.

It is this collection of fluid that can cause periods of rapid weight gain that some patients with heart failure experience.

Because it has to pump this greater volume of blood around the body, the main pumping chamber of the heart muscle (the left ventricle) gradually enlarges, which allows it to contract with greater force (a process that doctors call hypertrophy). But over time, this causes the muscle fibres in the ventricles to stretch, eventually leaving the heart with a larger, weaker ventricle that is not able to pump effectively, a condition that doctors call *left ventricular dysfunction*. This is the most frequent cause of heart failure.

How the heart gets damaged

Any disease that affects the heart and circulation can lead to damage and weakening of the heart muscle and ultimately to heart failure. In about 3 out of every 4 cases of heart failure, it is due to damage from *coronary heart disease*, a term that doctors use to describe the conditions that you probably know of as angina and heart attack.

Both angina and heart attacks occur when the coronary arteries – the arteries that deliver oxygen to the heart muscle – become narrowed over many years due to the build up of cholesterol from the food we eat. This process is called atherosclerosis, and leads to less oxygen being delivered to the heart muscle, which can reduce the ability of the heart to pump blood efficiently.

In some cases the coronary arteries become blocked by a blood clot that results in a heart attack. Modern medicines and emergency care have helped many millions of people to survive their heart attack and get back to a normal, active life. Unfortunately, for some people the heart attack leaves the heart muscle damaged, which can increase the chance of developing heart failure in the future.

Other causes of heart failure

Hypertension: Living with high blood pressure – or hypertension – can put a greater strain on the heart. Because the pressure in the circulatory system is higher, the heart has to pump harder in order to keep the same amount of blood flowing through the body. The heart responds to this extra workload by enlarging to provide a stronger contraction, but in time becomes strained as the muscle fibres within the ventricles stretch. Then they become less able to pump effectively. The chance of developing heart failure is higher if the hypertension is not picked up and treated properly.

Heart valve disease: In some people, heart failure may be caused by disease of the heart valves obstructing the blood flow between the chambers of the heart or between the heart and the major arteries. Alternatively, the valves may become leaky and less effective at keeping the blood pumping in the right direction, allowing blood to flow backwards.

In both cases, the result is that the heart has to work harder to pump enough blood around the body, and this increased workload eventually weakens the force of the contraction of the heart.

Congenital heart defects: Some people are born with abnormalities of the chambers or valves that increase the risk of the heart failing. The more severe the defect, the higher the risk of heart failure.

Heart rhythm disorders: In some people, heart failure may be caused by an abnormal and irregular heart rhythm, called atrial fibrillation.

Obesity: People who are very overweight are more likely to develop heart failure because the heart has to work harder to pump blood throughout a greater amount of body tissue. This puts strain on the heart and over the years increases the likelihood of the heart failing.

Diabetes: People with diabetes seem to have a stronger chance of developing heart failure. In part, this may be because diabetes is often associated with hypertension or coronary heart disease.

Other causes: In a few patients, weakening of the heart muscle may be due to infection, such as rheumatic fever, Chagas' disease, viruses (including Coxsackie or HIV), an overactive thyroid gland, poisoning by an excessive alcohol intake over months to years, or very rarely due to pregnancy.

Unknown causes: In some people the cause of the heart damage may not be clear – and the word 'cardiomyopathy' is used. In some cases this may be due to a problem with a gene, and this may run in families. Different terms are used to describe different types of 'cardiomyopathy' depending on how the heart is affected – 'dilated cardiomyopathy' if the heart chambers are enlarged, 'hypertrophic cardiomyopathy' if the heart muscle is very much thicker than normal, and 'restrictive cardiomyopathy' when the heart muscle is very stiff and doesn't relax properly.

Why it is important to know the cause of heart failure

It is important for doctors to find out the reason for the development of heart failure in each individual patient, as it may be possible to get rid of the heart failure if there is an underlying cause that can be remedied – such as heavy alcohol drinking, or a heart valve that can be replaced by an operation.

Also, the cause of heart failure may have a direct bearing upon the treatment that the patient receives.

Can heart failure be prevented?

Since many cases of heart failure are due to some form of underlying cardiovascular disease, development of heart failure can sometimes be prevented by early treatment of its underlying causes.

If you have angina or have had a heart attack, you should ask your doctor whether there is anything you should alter in your lifestyle to reduce your risk of developing further heart problems, including heart failure. This may involve taking tablets to lower your blood cholesterol level, stopping smoking, taking more exercise or losing some weight if you are overweight. If you have high blood pressure, you should be sure to take your tablets regularly to prevent your blood pressure putting undue strain on your heart.

How serious is heart failure?

Although in most cases there is no cure for heart failure, when it is diagnosed early enough the symptoms can be well controlled with medicines, diet and exercise. Your future outlook will depend on your age, the severity of your heart failure and your general health.

Your doctor will grade your heart failure as mild, moderate or severe, depending on the extent of your symptoms. If you have mild heart failure, you may have no symptoms at all, or they may appear only during physical activity. If your heart failure is more severe, the symptoms may become more apparent and may limit your ability to perform even simple every day activities such as housework or gardening. If you have severe heart failure, you may need to be admitted to hospital as an emergency. But the need for hospital admission can usually be avoided if you are given proper information about how to look after yourself, together with the right treatment.

Chapter 4

How will the doctor decide I have heart failure?

The most important aspect of diagnosing heart failure is recognising the symptoms and signs associated with the illness. Doctors are mainly interested in heart failure because it causes symptoms that can limit your quality of life and may shorten the length of your life – and correct treatment can make a big difference.

In the early stages of heart failure, you are most likely to feel tired and breathless when you do physical activity because your muscles are not getting an adequate amount of blood. If your heart failure is more severe, then you may notice fluid building up in your feet and ankles and breathlessness on gentle exertion. If the heart failure is severe, you will notice breathlessness even when you are doing nothing. The severity of the symptoms does not necessarily closely mirror the amount of underlying heart damage, and can change a lot from time to time, particularly in response to treatment.

Sometimes, if there is a lot of fluid building up in the lungs, you may wake up gasping for breath or wheezing. Sitting up will make the breathing easier, but you should notify your doctor or nurse if your condition has got worse as adjustment of your treatment can help alleviate all these symptoms.

There is a wide range of symptoms thought to be characteristic of heart failure. Depending on the severity of your illness, you may experience some or all of the following symptoms:

- Shortness of breath during physical activity, at night when lying in bed or all of the time
- Fatigue and weakness
- Swollen ankles and feet, and swelling of the legs, groin and abdomen
- Dry cough (this may also be a side effect of one of the tablets used to treat heart failure – the ACE inhibitors (see page 31)
- Dizzy spells
- Poor appetite, constipation, abdominal bloating

It is important to realise that many people, especially if they are unfit, putting on weight and getting older, feel breathless when they exercise more than is normal for them. These symptoms may not always be the result of heart failure – they may occur because we smoke or have lung diseases such as bronchitis, or perhaps because we are overweight. In some people, particularly in women, swelling of the legs may be the result of varicose veins or a side-effect of medicines. If you do have these symptoms it is important to see your doctor, who knows your medical history, can examine your heart and organise tests if necessary.

How is heart failure confirmed?

Before any of your symptoms can be assumed to be due to heart failure, your doctor needs proof that there is damage to your heart. He or she will discuss your symptoms with you and look at your medical history, and will also examine you. This will usually involve listening to your heart and taking your blood pressure. In addition, he or she will look for evidence of fluid in the lungs, legs and the rest of your body, and may organise a few blood tests to look for anaemia, diabetes, kidney damage or thyroid disease.

If the heart is not working properly, the muscle of the left ventricle of the heart becomes stretched and releases a hormone called *natriuretic peptide* into the blood. By analysing this protein in a blood sample doctors can now identify which patients are very unlikely to have heart failure. If your levels of natriuretic peptides are normal, then it is unlikely that there will have been any serious damage to your heart. But if you have high levels of these peptides then you are likely to have heart failure due to stretching of the left ventricle. So the blood test can indicate whether you need further investigation and possibly treatment.

Your doctor may also decide to send you to a heart failure clinic at the hospital for further tests: some tests will help in the diagnosis, some will help to assess how well your heart is performing and some will be carried out to determine the underlying cause of the heart failure – there may be something wrong that can be cured, rather than just treated. Your family doctor may be able to do some of these tests in the surgery rather than referring you to a clinic – this will vary from one area to another.

Electrocardiogram

An electrocardiogram (or ECG) is a simple test that picks up the electrical signals generated by your heart, amplifies them and records them on paper. The ECG is recorded by placing wire electrodes on your chest, arms and legs. These pick up the flow and direction of electric currents in your heart during each heartbeat.

By looking at your ECG recording, doctors can assess whether your heart rhythm and rate are normal; abnormalities may indicate whether there is any damage to the heart muscle perhaps due to a previous heart attack, or whether the heart is enlarged and thickened perhaps due to high blood pressure, which may be putting it under strain.

Although the ECG can provide useful information for your doctor, an ECG alone cannot provide enough evidence to diagnose heart failure. Other tests are needed too.

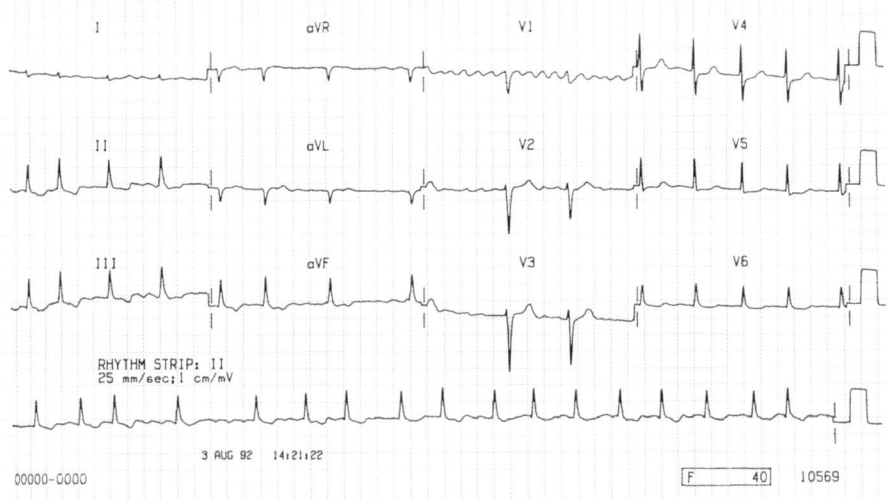

Figure 4.1. Electrocardiogram (ECG) of a patient with heart failure.

Chest X-ray

The chest X-ray shows the size of your heart and allows the doctor to decide whether it is enlarged, and whether the lungs are congested with fluid. Although a chest X-ray can be useful to the doctor, it cannot provide conclusive evidence for the presence of heart failure. Other tests are needed too. The chest X-ray may also show up a problem with the lungs rather than the heart.

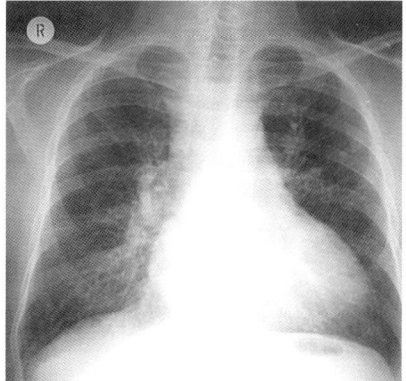

Figure 4.2. Chest X-ray of a patient with heart failure showing a large heart (in centre) and fluid in the lungs (either side of heart).

Echocardiogram

An echocardiogram is a sound wave test that produces a picture of the structure and movement of your heart. This is produced by bouncing very high frequency sound waves off the wall of your heart. A sound probe placed on the chest picks up the echoes that are bounced back from your heart. Moving the probe around allows the doctor to visualise (usually on a video screen) the different parts of your heart and its valves. In this way the doctor can 'see' how effectively your heart is pumping blood and whether there is any damage to the heart muscle. This test is completely painless and works on the same principle as the scan that a pregnant women has to look at the child in the womb – although this time it is the heart that is the object of interest.

Echocardiography is probably the best and simplest way to confirm the doctor's suspicion of heart failure. Because the echocardiogram can show which part of the heart is not able to pump properly and also how well the heart valves are working, it will often help the doctor to get a pretty good idea of what has caused your heart failure.

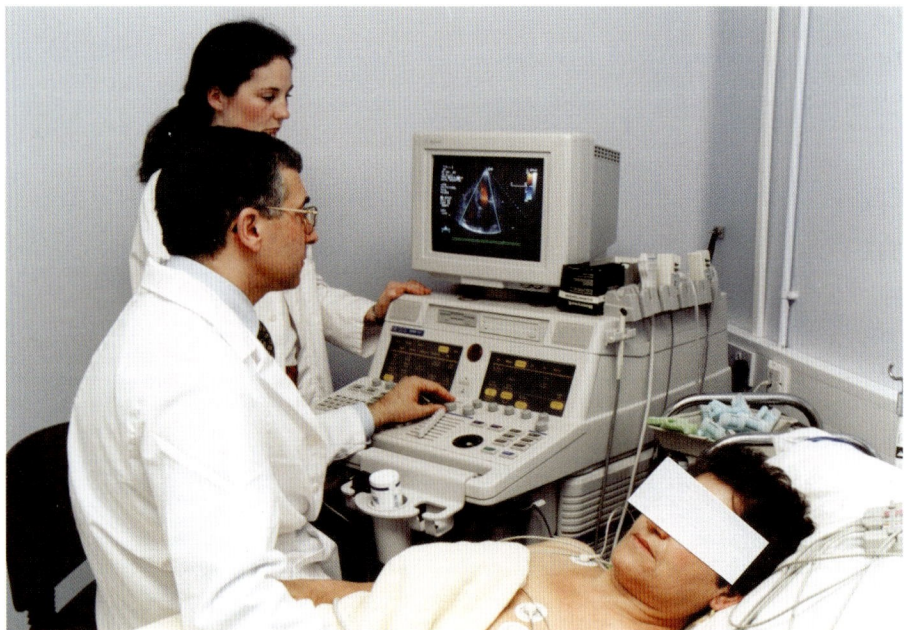

Figure 4.3. Patient undergoing echocardiogram.

Exercise testing

An exercise test – sometimes called a stress test – can reveal problems that are not apparent when you are resting. It involves continuously monitoring the ECG and blood pressure while you undertake exercise, usually at a set pace on a treadmill. As you exercise, the doctor will monitor you for symptoms, such as shortness of breath or chest pain, and will stop the test if these become too uncomfortable.

Although an exercise test is not usually used to diagnose heart failure, it may be used to assess the seriousness of the heart failure and to help select the right treatment.

Lung function tests

The doctor may decide to perform some tests that measure how well and how deeply you are able to breathe. Although these tests are not so useful for diagnosing heart failure, they are useful in ruling out other respiratory causes for your breathlessness, such as bronchitis or emphysema.

Cardiac catheterisation

The pumping efficiency of the heart and abnormalities of the chambers, valves and coronary arteries can be examined using cardiac catheterisation. Under local anaesthesia, a long, thin tube called a catheter will be inserted through an artery or vein – usually in your arm or leg – and guided to the heart chambers using an X-ray machine. When it reaches your heart, a colourless dye will be injected into the heart's blood supply through the catheter. Under an X-ray, this dye shows whether there are any narrowings in your coronary arteries, and can also show any problems with pumping or with the valves of the heart.

Although cardiac catheterisation is not usually used to diagnose heart failure, it may be used to identify the cause of the heart failure and to assess its seriousness. In a very few cases, where the cause of the heart failure is unclear, cardiac catheterisation may be used to obtain a small piece of heart muscle tissue for microscopic examination (biopsy).

What other illnesses might be identified in patients with heart failure?

In all the tests that the doctors perform, they will be looking for other illnesses that might be contributing to your heart failure and which, if treated, might relieve your symptoms.

In particular, the doctors will be looking to see whether you have other diseases that may affect the doctor's diagnosis and choice of treatment for you, such as kidney or liver disease, lung disease or thyroid disease.

If you have high blood pressure you'll be advised to keep it under control, usually by means of drugs. Similarly, if you have diabetes, you'll be advised about how important it is to keep your blood sugar levels under control, by watching what you eat and if necessary by taking tablets.

If you have high cholesterol levels (hyperlipidaemia), then you may be advised to take tablets that will help to lower them, especially if you also have other symptoms of coronary heart disease such as angina.

If the tests show a problem with your heart rate or rhythm, then the doctor will organise further tests such as a 24-hour recording of your heart rhythm (Holter recording). Some patients will then require a change in their medications, or your doctor may recommend an artificial pacemaker or an implantable defibrillator [see section on treatments in next chapter].

What happens after all the tests?

If the tests confirm that you have heart failure, then your symptoms may be used to classify the severity of your illness. This will allow your doctor to monitor your condition. It will help your doctor if you can describe what makes you breathless, and whether this has improved, got worse or stayed the same since your last check up. Remember, your symptoms may fluctuate from one day to another, but a steady worsening needs to be brought to your doctor's attention as soon as possible.

One of the most commonly used classification systems is the New York Heart Association rating scale (see panel opposite).

Your doctor will use this classification system to decide which treatments might be suitable for you and will devise a treatment programme to achieve three aims:

- to treat your heart failure
- to treat the underlying cause of your heart failure
- to remove the factors that may cause your heart failure to worsen.

Treatment may involve taking drugs or, in some cases, undergoing surgery. These are explained in the next chapter.

In general, being in the more severe classes of heart failure is associated with a greater chance of further problems with your heart, so it is safer to

The New York Heart Association classification of heart failure	
Class	Definition
Class I	Ordinary physical exercise does not cause undue fatigue or breathlessness
Class II	Slight limitation of physical activity: comfortable at rest but ordinary physical activity, for example minor activities such as climbing a flight of stairs, getting dressed or doing housework results in fatigue, palpitations or breathlessness
Class III	Marked limitation of physical activity: comfortable at rest but symptoms such as breathlessness occur when walking on a flat surface
Class IV	Unable to carry out any physical activity without discomfort: symptoms occur even at rest with increased discomfort with any physical activity

be in the less severe classes. The good news is that by taking the right treatments and managing your lifestyle in the right way, you can reduce the symptoms and their impact on your day-to-day life. You will also be much less likely to require a period in hospital. If, however, your symptoms do deteriorate your doctor (or heart failure nurse) will be able to work with you to help improve things again.

Chapter 5

How is heart failure treated?

The best way of treating heart failure is to prevent it occurring in the first place, or to reverse the underlying cause of heart damage as early as possible. This is not always possible. Fortunately, in recent years there have been some important advances in treatment using medicines that have been shown to prolong life and to improve the quality of life for people with heart failure. Some people, however, may need surgery to help their condition. This chapter outlines the various types of drugs available for the treatment of heart failure and the operations that might be undertaken depending on the underlying cause of the illness. Your doctor will be able to tell you which treatments are likely to benefit you.

What drugs will I be given?

If the tests show that you have heart failure, then your doctors will offer you treatment using several different types of drugs. The major types of drugs used to treat heart failure are shown in the table. Not all people with heart failure require all of these drugs – but most will take a 'diuretic' (water tablet), an 'ACE inhibitor' and a 'beta-blocker'. All tablets have side-effects, and these will be explained by your doctor or heart failure nurse. Your medication will come in a packet with written information about all the possible side-effects but it is important you realise that not everyone who takes a tablet will get the side-effects listed. The doctors and nurses advising you will monitor you for possible side-effects, and will arrange to check various blood tests from time to time.

Before buying any medicines 'over the counter' at a chemist's shop, you should tell the pharmacist you have heart failure and let him or her know what tablets you are taking. This will ensure that you do not take drugs that might worsen your condition, or react with your heart failure medicines.

How is heart failure treated?

Major drugs used in treatment of chronic heart failure

Drug	Purpose	Examples	Major side-effects*
Thiazide diuretics	To help remove excess fluid from the body	Bendrofluazide Hydrochlorothiazide	Hypokalaemia, hyponatraemia (upset balance of salts in the blood)
Loop diuretics		Frusemide Bumetanide Torasemide	Hypokalaemia, hyponatraemia May worsen control of sugar levels in diabetes, light-headedness
Potassium-sparing diuretics		Amiloride Triamterene Spironolactone (Aldactone)	Hyperkalaemia, rash Hyperkalaemia, gynaecomastia (tender enlargement of the breasts, usually more of a problem in men)
ACE inhibitors	To make it easier for the heart to pump, to increase the amount of blood pumped and to improve symptoms of heart failure	Captopril (Capoten) Enalapril (Innovace) Lisinopril (Zestril) Quinapril (Accupro) Perindopril (Coversyl) Ramipril (Tritace) Cilazapril (Vascace) Fosinopril (Staril) Trandolapril (Gopten)	Dry cough, light-headedness
Angiotensin II receptor antagonists	To make it easier for the heart to pump, to increase the amount of blood pumped and to improve symptoms of heart failure	Losartan (Cozaar) Valsartan (Diovan) Irbesartan (Aprovel) Candesartan (Amias) Telmisartan (Micardis) Eprosartan (Teveten)	Light-headedness
Beta-blockers	To slow the heart rate, and to help the heart pump better	Carvedilol (Eucardic) Bisoprolol (Cardicor) Metoprolol (Betaloc)	Tiredness, light-headeness, wheeze
Cardiac glycosides	To strengthen the heart muscle and control the irregular heart beat of atrial fibrillation	Digoxin (Lanoxin)	Nausea, vomiting

*Not everyone taking these tablets will experience these side-effects. You should report any change in symptoms on taking medication, particularly if it is a new medication, to your doctor or heart failure nurse.

Diuretics

Diuretics are the first drugs that patients with heart failure suffering from symptoms of fluid retention (especially lung congestion and swollen ankles) are likely to be given. They are usually taken by mouth, but in emergency cases they can be given by injection into a vein.

Diuretics are more commonly known as 'water tablets'; they will make your kidneys produce more urine, which will remove sodium and water from the body. This may reduce your blood pressure as well as the amount of fluid circulating in your body, which in turn reduces the amount of work your heart has to do. As a result, there is an improvement in the symptoms of heart failure, especially ankle swelling and breathlessness.

You should avoid taking too much salt in your food as this can make the diuretics less effective.

Also, you will probably be asked to keep a daily record of your weight. This can be useful in helping your doctor or heart failure nurse to adjust the dose of your diuretics in order to ensure that you do not either become severely overloaded with fluid, or too dehydrated.

Commonly used diuretics include the 'thiazides', such as bendrofluazide and hydrochlorothiazide, and 'loop' diuretics such as frusemide, bumetanide and torasemide. Unfortunately, these can cause the body to lose potassium, so the doctor will probably arrange for a blood test if you are started on one of these diuretics. If potassium is being lost, then a potassium-sparing diuretic such as amiloride may be added. Alternatively, you may be given a diuretic called spironolactone (Aldactone). This is a drug that has been shown to reduce symptoms and increase life expectancy in patients with the more advanced stages of heart failure.

If you go on holiday to a warmer place than you are used to, you may lose more salt and water in perspiration and therefore need a smaller dose of diuretic than you are used to. Your doctor will advise you about this, and monitoring your weight may be a good way of keep your diuretic medication at the correct level.

ACE inhibitors and angiotensin II receptor antagonists

A group of drugs called angiotensin converting enzyme (ACE) inhibitors have been shown not only to improve symptoms in patients with heart failure but also to prolong life. They are of particular benefit if the heart failure is due to abnormalities in how well the left ventricle (the major pumping chamber of the heart) pumps.

ACE inhibitors block the body's production of a substance called angiotensin II, which has been shown to make blood vessels contract. By causing your blood vessels to relax, ACE inhibitors make it easier for your heart to pump blood through them, which is why they are commonly also used as a treatment for hypertension (high blood pressure). This, in turn, reduces the amount of work your heart has to do, and so helps to relieve heart failure. If your heart has become enlarged, then treatment with an ACE inhibitor may well help your heart to return to normal size.

However, as with all drugs, some people develop side-effects when treated with an ACE inhibitor. In some people they can cause kidney damage, although this is rare. The most commonly experienced side-effect of ACE inhibitors is an irritating dry cough. If this develops, your doctor can prescribe an alternative drug from a class called the 'angiotensin II receptor antagonists.' These are a good second choice and have similar effects but without the troublesome cough.

Commonly used ACE inhibitors include enalapril (Innovace), captopril (Capoten), fosinopril (Staril), lisinopril (Zestril), ramipril (Tritace), perindopril (Coversyl) and quinapril (Accupro). Commonly used angiotensin II antagonists include valsartan (Diovan), losartan (Cozaar), irbesartan (Aprovel), candesartan (Amias), telmisartan (Micardis) and eprosartan (Teveten).

Beta-blockers

Beta-blockers are effective drugs that slow the heart beat and reduce the amount of work your heart has to do. Some, such as carvedilol (Eucardic), also relax the blood vessels, which makes it easier for the heart to pump blood through them. Beta-blockers are often given to patients with high blood pressure or angina, but for patients with heart failure the starting dose is much smaller, and the dose is only gradually increased in small steps to the final dose which is similar to that used for the treatment of the other conditions.

In patients with heart failure, beta-blockers are thought to block the excessive stimulation that commonly occurs in the failing heart. They have been shown not only to improve symptoms but also to prolong life when given to patients who have evidence of damage to the pumping of the left ventricle and who are already taking diuretics and ACE inhibitors. But in order to avoid lowering blood pressure too much and causing other symptoms to emerge, it is important to get the beta-blocker dose exactly right. This means starting at a low dose and increasing it gradually over several weeks. For this reason, the introduction of beta-blockers and the increase in dosage is often monitored by a specialist heart failure nurse.

Like most drugs, beta-blockers can have side-effects: they can make you feel tired, and may give you cold hands and feet. Beta-blockers can also cause the airways to narrow, so they should be avoided in people who have asthma, bronchitis or other lung problems.

Beta-blockers can cause impotence in some men. If you find that you are unable to get an erection, then you should speak to your doctor, as it may be possible for an alternative medication to be prescribed.

Beta-blockers commonly used in patients with heart failure include carvedilol (Eucardic) or bisoprolol (Cardicor).

Cardiac glycosides

Cardiac glycosides such as digoxin (Lanoxin) are the oldest known treatments for heart failure, having been used since at least the 18th century when it was found that an extract from the foxglove plant was able to stimulate the heart in people who had 'dropsy' caused by heart disease.

Digoxin increases the power of the heart beat and slows the heart rate, particularly if it is irregular. If you are given digoxin, it is probably because you also have an irregular heart rhythm called atrial fibrillation. Digoxin has been shown to reduce the likelihood of heart failure patients with atrial fibrillation requiring admission to hospital.

Side-effects of digoxin treatment may include nausea and vomiting, diarrhoea, confusion and hallucinations. Other medications can affect the levels of digoxin in your body, so it is particularly important that you tell your pharmacist (and remind your doctor) that you are taking this medication should you need other tablets.

Keep taking the tablets

Whatever drugs you are given for your heart failure, it is important that you keep taking them at the doses and times recommended by your doctor or heart failure specialist nurse. Following the right advice will ensure that your tablets help you to live a longer and more active life.

If you find it difficult to remember to take your tablets at the correct times, then speak with your doctor or the pharmacist in your local chemist shop. They will be able to suggest ways of making it easier for you to remember. Sometimes, this can be as easy as linking your medicine-taking with everyday routines such as eating breakfast or brushing your teeth. In some cases, the pharmacist may be able to help by putting your tablets in a weekly pill box.

It is important you do not suddenly stop taking your medication. You should contact your family doctor in plenty of time to get a repeat prescription. If you are going on holiday you should take sufficient medication to last you through your stay (and a little longer in case you experience delay in returning home).

Can heart failure be treated by surgery?

For some patients, it may be possible to correct heart failure symptoms by surgery, particularly if the doctor has identified a distinct underlying cause for the symptoms that can be rectified by surgery.

There are three main situations in which you may be advised to consider having an operation:

- If your heart failure is due to coronary heart disease and if you have angina (chest pain when you exert yourself) then you may be offered a procedure to replumb the blood supply to the heart – either by an angioplasty (an operation done under a local anaesthetic in which a small balloon is used at the time of cardiac catheterisation to relieve obstructions in the blood vessels supplying the heart muscle) or by open heart surgery (a bypass operation). [See section on revascularisation for further details]

- If your heart failure is due to a damaged heart valve, it may be possible to have an operation to repair or replace the faulty heart valve.

- If your heart failure is severe and is not being controlled by drug treatments, then you may be eligible for heart transplantation. However, in general, this is only likely to be an option for a very limited number of patients: the number of donor hearts available is limited and it is only really suitable for patients who are fit and strong enough to cope with the rigours of undergoing this major procedure and the close follow-up necessary after the operation.

Your family doctor will need to refer you to see a specialist (usually a cardiologist or cardiac surgeon) for a full assessment before you would be advised to have an operation. More recently, doctors have found that some patients with coronary heart disease but no angina may benefit from a bypass operation. Your specialist will consider whether this is likely to be the case for you – and may order some further tests before advising you about this.

Revascularisation

Coronary revascularisation is a means of treating blocked coronary arteries, so that they are once again able to deliver oxygen and nutrients to the heart muscle. Arteries often become narrowed as cholesterol and fats build up on their inner lining over many years.

How is heart failure treated?

There are two types of revascularisation operations: percutaneous transluminal coronary angioplasty (or balloon angioplasty) and coronary artery bypass grafting (CABG).

Balloon angioplasty is a non-surgical procedure carried out under a local anaesthetic. A long, thin tube called a catheter will be inserted into an artery in your groin or your arm. From there it is guided by means of an X-ray machine to the blocked section of the coronary artery by the cardiologist who watches the X-ray pictures on a TV monitor.

A tiny balloon at the end of the catheter is then inflated (usually up to a diameter of about 3 mm), flattening the mass of fatty tissue blocking the artery against the wall of the artery. Usually, a short tube of stainless steel mesh called a stent is inserted into the artery to help keep it open and to prevent it from narrowing again. After a minute or so, the balloon is deflated and the catheter is removed, leaving the artery unblocked so the blood can flow freely again.

Most patients are able to go home the day after an angioplasty; most are back to their normal activity within 3-4 days.

Bypass grafting is a major operation that is carried out under a general anaesthetic. It usually involves opening up the chest by cutting through the breastbone. A vein or artery will be taken from somewhere else in your body (usually from the chest or the leg) and joined (or grafted) between the main artery leaving the heart (the aorta) and some point beyond the narrowed or blocked coronary artery. Several narrowings can be bypassed at the same operation. While it is being performed, the heart is stopped and a heart-lung bypass machine maintains the circulation. This breathes for you, making sure that the blood flow to the brain and the rest of the body is not interrupted.

Like any operation, bypass surgery carries risks. These will depend on your age and any other medical conditions you may have; before you decide to go ahead with the operation, your surgeon will discuss these risks with you.

You'll probably have to stay in hospital for 7–10 days after your bypass operation. As it is a major operation, you may not recover fully until 2–3 months later, as the wound takes time to heal. During that time you may be invited to take part in a cardiac rehabilitation programme that will include regular exercise sessions and advice on healthy eating and relaxation techniques.

Valve surgery

The heart contains valves that ensure that blood always flows in the right direction. If the valves are diseased or damaged, they may not close or open properly. This means the heart has to work harder to pump blood around the body, which puts an extra strain on the heart muscle.

Doctors can diagnose *valvular heart disease* by listening to the heart (see chapter 2) and looking at the state of the valves through tests such as echocardiography. In some cases, if the valve is leaking but is not seriously damaged, it is possible to repair it. If it is more seriously damaged, the valve may be replaced altogether, usually with a metal or plastic valve, or a 'tissue' valve, whether from a human or an animal (usually a pig or a cow).

Valve surgery is a major operation, carried out under a general anaesthetic. It involves opening up the chest by cutting through the breastbone. In order to keep the body supplied with fresh blood while the surgeon operates, the blood circulation will be diverted from the heart and the lungs by a heart-lung bypass machine. In effect, this machine breathes for you. The surgeon is then able to open up the heart to repair the damaged valve or replace it.

If the new valve is made from an artificial material there is a chance of a blood clot forming on the new valve or inside the heart chambers. The surgeons will try to guard against this by giving you a blood-thinning (anticoagulant) medicine such as warfarin. You may also need to take warfarin for a few weeks after a tissue valve replacement. Anticoagulants reduce the chance of blood clots forming, but it is important to get the dose right as taking too much can lead to bleeding problems. This will involve regular blood tests, usually at the anticoagulant clinic of the local hospital or at your doctor's surgery. If you are on warfarin, you must make sure you do not take any additional medication without your doctor or pharmacist being aware of this – you may need to adjust your normal dose of warfarin and/or have more frequent blood tests to check that your dose is still appropriate for you.

Like any operation, valve surgery carries risks. These will depend on your age and any other medical conditions you may have; before you decide to go ahead with the operation, your surgeon will discuss these risks with you.

Heart transplantation

In theory, heart transplantation may be an option for patients whose heart failure is no longer effectively controlled by drug treatment and whose heart is so severely damaged that they are at high risk of dying.

Only a limited number are done each year – usually about 300 – in this country. This compares to around 65,000 people developing heart failure each year. Not all of these people, of course, need a heart transplant.

Patients who are generally not suitable for heart transplantation
- Patients who misuse alcohol or recreational drugs
- Patients who have been treated for cancer within the past 5 years
- Patients with other diseases that affect many body organs
- Patients with uncontrolled infection
- Patients with severe kidney disease
- Patients who have recently had leg ulcers or deep vein thrombosis
- Patients with an unhealed peptic ulcer
- Patients with evidence of significant liver damage
- Patients with other disease with a poor life expectancy

Not all patients are suitable for heart transplantation (see table), but if your cardiologist thinks you may benefit from a transplant, you will be referred to one of these centres for a specialist assessment. Whether or not you are suitable will depend on:

- what other illnesses you have
- whether or not your kidneys are in good working order
- whether or not you are fit enough to undergo the operation.

The doctors at the transplant centre will decide whether or not to put you on the waiting list for a transplant should a suitable heart become available: the number of transplants offered is severely limited by the availability of donor hearts.

If a suitable donor heart becomes available you could be called to go in for your operation at any time, although most people have to wait for around 6 months. If your condition is serious enough you may have to stay in hospital while you are waiting.

As soon as a suitable donor heart is available, you will be taken into the transplant centre and examined again to make sure that there is nothing wrong that might affect the success of the operation.

As a major operation, which may take as long as 5 hours, transplantation is carried out under a general anaesthetic. The surgeon will cut through the breastbone to open the chest. As with valvular surgery, the blood circulation will be diverted from your heart and the lungs by a heart-lung machine that will, in effect, breathe for you and make sure that the blood flow to your brain and the rest of your body is not interrupted. Having isolated your damaged heart, the surgeon will then replace it with the donor heart.

After the operation, you will remain on a ventilator in the intensive care unit for some time. Once you have improved, you will be moved to a special ward where the medical staff can protect you from any kind of infection. Here, you'll be given drugs to prevent your body from rejecting your new heart; you may have to continue to take some of these drugs for several months or even years after your operation.

Two or 3 weeks after the operation, you will be discharged from hospital, but it will still be several months before you start getting back to a normal way of life. To help you do so, you will probably be invited to join a cardiac rehabilitation programme that will provide you with exercise and physiotherapy, as well as information about how to live with your new heart and how to prevent developing any new problems related to it. You will also need to have specialist check ups at regular intervals after your discharge from hospital.

Other treatments for heart rhythm disorders

Some patients may require treatments for problems with their heart rhythm. This may include drugs, but may also include an artificial pacemaker or an implantable defibrillator.

An **artificial pacemaker** is usually fitted for people who have a very slow heart rhythm. The pacemaker consists of a power supply that generates a pulse, and a lead that delivers an electrical impulse to the chambers of your heart. The whole unit is very small and is fitted in a small pouch under the skin of your chest. Fitting a pacemaker takes around an hour under a local anaesthetic, but you will usually need to stay in hospital overnight. You will need pacemaker checks afterwards – usually each year. The batteries will last for 5–10 years before needing to be replaced.

An **implantable defibrillator** may be offered to people who have attacks of very fast heart beat, which may cause them to pass out or cause the heart to stop pumping. This is a small device that is usually fitted under the skin and is connected to your heart by a wire that will be passed through a vein. The defibrillator will monitor the rhythm of your heart and give out a strong electrical signal if your heart starts beating too fast. This signal reverts the heart to its normal rhythm. Fitting a defibrillator usually involves a 2–3 day stay in hospital for the operation, which is usually carried out under a local anaesthetic. The defibrillator will need regular checks afterwards.

Chapter 6

How will treatment affect my everyday life?

In addition to treating your heart failure and its underlying causes, your doctor will need you to play an important part in helping to remove the factors that may worsen your heart failure. This will go a long way towards helping you to be able to undertake everyday physical activities with little difficulty and to live with a very much improved quality of life.

Get to know your heart failure nurse

In many illnesses, once you have been seen by the doctor and given your tablets you are left to get better on your own. It's not like that in heart failure.

Once you have started on a treatment programme, you will usually continue to receive follow-up care from your GP or heart failure nurse. The ongoing contact with these health care professionals is one of the most important aspects of care in heart failure.

The heart failure nurse is a good source of general help and advice both for you and for the other members of your family. He or she will help you to understand what heart failure is and why symptoms occur, how to recognise symptoms and what to do if they occur.

In addition, your heart failure nurse will be able to help you cope with some of the more difficult aspects of living with heart failure.

Heart failure, even when it is treated, can seriously affect your quality of life and your attitudes towards life. It is not uncommon for people to get depressed. If you find your condition gets you down, you shouldn't just suffer in silence – talk to your heart failure nurse or your doctor as there are ways they can help you.

As part of your treatment plan, your heart failure nurse or your doctor may also be able to help you to decide whether you need long-term social support, for example, a home help. The nurse or your GP will have links with Social Services and may be able to put you in touch with the right people.

They may also be able to help you to contact a patient support group. You can find details of how to contact these groups in the section at the end of this book.

But because there are several changes that you may need to make to your lifestyle, helping you to understand what you need to do and why is probably one of the most important ways in which the heart failure nurse will be able to help you. These changes are geared towards helping to remove the things that make your heart failure symptoms worse, such as smoking, eating too much salt, being overweight and drinking too much alcohol. These are outlined in this chapter.

What do I have to do about my diet?

The most important dietary adjustment that you'll need to make is to cut down the amount of salt you take. Salt causes the body to retain fluid. Taking in too much salt will counteract the effect of the diuretics that you will have been given. Remember, diuretics will generally make you pass water more often, and so will help to reduce symptoms of fluid retention.

The simplest way to reduce the amount of salt in your diet is to avoid adding salt to your meals at the table, to cook with less salt (try using spices instead), and to avoid buying salted foods such as peanuts and snacks and products like soy sauce. You should also try to avoid, or cut down on, processed meats such as salami, and ready-made convenience meals, as these tend to contain a lot of salt.

Since you really need to stop your body retaining too much fluid, it will also help if you can cut down on the amount of fluids that you take in. Try to limit your water intake to between 2 and 3 pints a day (unless the weather gets very hot). Don't forget that drinks such as tea and coffee are mostly water, but they also contain caffeine, which increases urination. Your doctor or heart failure nurse will tell you whether or not you should avoid them.

Watch your weight

Watching your weight every day is a simple and reliable way of checking whether your body is retaining excess fluid. Your doctor or heart failure nurse will probably give you a chart to fill in so you have a record of your daily weight. It is best to weigh yourself at the same time every morning, on the same set of weighing scales, after going to the toilet but before you get dressed and have breakfast.

If your weight starts to rise quickly by more than about 3–5 pounds in a week, this will almost certainly be because your body is holding on to too much water. If the weight gain is consistent, then your heart failure may be getting worse. You should tell your doctor or heart failure nurse as soon as possible, as they may be able to adjust the dose of your drugs, or add in another drug to help the situation.

Try to eat more healthily

Following the advice above on salt and water will certainly help to reduce symptoms of fluid retention such as ankle swelling. But you should also try to follow a healthier diet, as this has been shown to reduce the chance of developing further heart and circulatory diseases.

As well as helping you to feel better, eating more healthily may also help you to lose weight if you need to. The best way to start is to try to eat less fat by opting for fish, lean meat and poultry rather than red meat and using low fat cheeses and spreads rather than full-fat cheese and butter, and to eat more high fibre foods such as wholemeal bread, pasta, fruit and vegetables. In between meals, you should try to eat fewer biscuits, sweets and chocolates.

Drink in moderation

Although there is evidence to suggest that alcohol is good for the heart and the circulatory system, it is sensible to limit your intake of alcohol to 1 or 2 units per day at most. Alcohol is not only very high in calories it is also likely to lead you to forget your good intentions regarding your diet!

Importantly, alcohol is actually very harmful in some patients with heart failure. If your heart failure was brought on by alcohol in the first place,

Try to eat more:	Try to eat less:
√ Fresh vegetables and salad	X High fat foods
√ Fresh fruit	X Butter, cream and cheese
√ Fresh fish	X Full fat milk
√ Fresh poultry (chicken and turkey)	X Cakes and biscuits
√ Lean meat	X Sweets
√ Wholemeal bread	X Snacks (especially crisps and peanuts, which are high in salt)
√ Cereals	
√ Starchy foods (such as potatoes and pasta)	X Salty foods (such as bacon, salami and other processed meats, cheese, corned beef, ham, pizza, sausages, salad dressings, tinned soups, ready-made meals)
√ Skimmed or semi-skimmed milk	

then your doctor will tell you to avoid alcohol altogether, even if your heart has recovered. If you start drinking again it is almost inevitable that your heart will be damaged again.

Try to stay active

Be careful that you don't pay too much attention to the old idea that when you feel ill you go to bed to recover. Staying in bed may be necessary in some situations, but as a rule, if your heart failure is stable then you should remain as active as possible.

That's because taking gentle physical activity is very good for the heart, the circulation and your muscles, provided you don't overdo it. Most people feel better when they exercise regularly but you should talk to your doctor or heart failure nurse first. He or she will be able to give you some advice about how much exercise you should do, and of what type. It is important to avoid activities that require you to hold your breath, lift heavy weights or (if you also suffer from angina) cause symptoms such as chest pain. Remember, you want to avoid too much stress. The golden rule is, don't do any form of exercise that makes you very breathless.

That means that no one will suggest you take out an expensive gym membership: brisk walking, golfing or swimming, or even walking down to the shops or gardening all count as physical activity, although some people find taking up bowls or line dancing to be more interesting!

Stub out the cigarettes

Smoking is generally very harmful to the heart and is linked to the development of heart disease. In patients with heart failure it tends to make the blood vessels in the body contract and increases the amount of oxygen that they require while at the same time reducing the amount of blood that the heart is able to pump while also increasing the heart rate and blood pressure.

So patients with heart failure are usually encouraged to give it up.

Stopping smoking is not easy, but your GP can now help you, for instance by prescribing nicotine replacement therapy in the form of patches, gum, tablets or nasal sprays.

Often, people find it helpful to set a date (not too far away) on which they plan to quit smoking. It helps to get your family and friends involved, especially to make sure that they are not going to smoke in front of you!

Try to avoid going to places where you usually buy cigarettes, or places and situations in which you usually smoke. You'll find that many GP surgeries now run smoking cessation clinics, where you can get practical help and support to help you kick the habit.

Avoid infections

Getting 'flu and chest infections can make anyone feel pretty bad, but they are far worse if you have heart failure. You should consider getting immunised against influenza every autumn, and possibly against other infections such as pneumococcal pneumonia. Your GP or practice nurse will be able to tell you when you should get your jabs.

If you have had a heart valve repaired or replaced, you will need to take antibiotics before having dental or other surgery in order to avoid the risk of infections. You should be given a card to carry that tells your dentist what antibiotics you require.

Don't forget the tablets

Heart failure is a long-term illness. To stand the best chance of keeping your symptoms under control and staying out of hospital, you really need to keep taking your medicines at the doses and times recommended by your doctor or heart failure specialist nurse.

But it's not easy. Remembering to take 5 or 6 different tablets each day can be difficult and there will always be times when something will make you forget to take them, maybe because you are away from home for a few days or somebody comes to stay and your normal routines become disturbed.

Medicines checklist

- Make sure you take your medicines every day, even if you are unwell
- Always have a good supply of your medicines – make sure you arrange for your repeat prescription before you run out of tablets
- Take all your tablets with you on your clinic visits to show to the doctor or heart failure nurse
- Keep taking the tablets until your doctor or heart failure nurse tells you to stop
- If you develop any side-effects from taking your medicines, don't simply stop taking the tablets – always talk to the doctor or heart failure nurse first
- Remember, taking your medicines is the best way to prevent your heart failure getting any worse
- If you are taking any medicines for conditions other than heart failure (maybe aspirin, heartburn or cold remedies) tell your doctor or heart failure nurse

If you miss a dose of one or more of your tablets, don't take more tablets to make up for the missed doses. Just start again with your next scheduled dose and talk to your heart failure nurse. He or she may be able to suggest ways to help make sure you don't miss your tablets.

If you experience problematic or unpleasant side-effects from your tablets, the heart failure nurse can advise you on how to manage these.

Remember, the reason for taking your tablets is that they will help you to live a longer and more enjoyable life.

Be careful about other drugs you are taking

Some of the drugs you may be taking for other conditions can cause your body to retain fluid, which is of course one of the actions that your heart failure drugs are designed to counteract. These include certain painkillers called non-steroidal anti-inflammatory drugs, which you may be taking for rheumatism, and corticosteroid tablets (but not inhalers), which you may be taking for asthma or other conditions.

In addition, some drugs do not react well when taken at the same time as the drugs you will have been given for your heart failure. Taking non-steroidal anti-inflammatory drugs or lithium at the same time as heart

Drugs that may affect your heart failure medicines

- Non-steroidal anti-inflammatory painkillers including ibuprofen (Nurofen)
- Certain drugs used to treat heart rhythm problems (especially quinidine and flecainide)
- Some medication used to treat high blood pressure or angina (especially verapamil, diltiazem, nifedipine)
- Some of the older-fashioned antidepressants (such as imipramine, amitriptyline, clomipramine, dothiepin, lofepramine or nortriptyline)
- Corticosteroids such as prednisolone
- Lithium

failure drugs can cause problems with the kidney, so you should make sure that your doctor or heart failure nurse knows if you are taking any of these drugs, or are prescribed one by another doctor.

Travelling with heart failure

Many patients with heart failure worry about whether or not they are able to go on holiday or to travel abroad. In most cases there is no reason why you should not but it is a good idea to talk through your travel plans with your doctor or heart failure nurse.

In general, holidaying at high altitudes or to very hot or humid places is not advisable. Short air flights are preferable to long journeys by other forms of transport. Don't be afraid to ask for help at the airport, especially if you have to walk a long distance to your plane. If you have severe heart failure, long air flights can cause you to become dehydrated, or other problems such as excessive limb swelling or deep venous thrombosis. Also, don't forget that changes in diet on journeys may upset your stomach.

If you are travelling to hot humid climates, you may need to adapt your dosage of diuretics and other drugs to avoid losing too much fluid. Again, your doctor or heart failure nurse will be able to give you good advice.

Can I still have sex?

There is no reason why you should not still enjoy an active sex life just because you have heart failure.

One important point to remember is that however worried you are about whether or not having sex is safe for you, the chances are that your partner will be even more worried! Your doctor or heart failure nurse may be able to help put both your minds at rest. Some drugs used to treat heart failure can cause impotence – if this is a problem you should mention this to your doctor or nurse.

Watch for the signs of worsening heart failure

Call your doctor or heart failure nurse if:

- You notice your breathing becoming more difficult
- You become short of breath when you are lying down or wake up at night short of breath
- You gain more than about 3–5 lbs in a week
- Your feet, ankles or stomach begin to become swollen
- You develop any side-effects from your tablets

Dial 999 and ask for an ambulance if:

- You become extremely short of breath
- You have tightness or pain in your chest for the first time or if you have an angina attack that does not go away after 20 minutes

It's your illness – take control of it

Taking an active part in your own treatment can help to improve your heart failure. As far as possible, you should try to become knowledgeable about your disease and its symptoms, as well as about the medicines you are taking for it and about the side-effects they may cause. Taking control of your heart failure also means learning about what foods you should and should not eat and about what activities should be limited.

You'll find it may help to write down a list of all your medicines and the instructions you have been given about taking them by your doctor or heart failure nurse.

Try to develop your own daily medicines schedule to make sure that you don't miss a dose. Also, you should keep a record of any weight you gain or lose and of any symptoms you develop.

Appendix

Sources of help and information

There are many organisations that offer help, support and information to people living with heart failure. You may find some of the following helpful

British Cardiac Patients Association

Unit 5D 2 Station Road
Swavesey
Cambridge CB4 5QJ
Tel/Fax: 01954 202022; National Helpline: 01223 846845
www.cardiac-bcpa.co.uk

British Heart Foundation

14 Fitzhardinge Street
London W1H 4DH
Tel: 0207 487 9419; Fax: 0207 486 1273
www.bhf.org.uk

Cardiomyopathy Association

40 The Metro Centre
Tolpits Lane
Watford
Herts WD1 8SB
Tel: 01923 249 977; Fax: 01923 249 987
Freephone: 0800 018 1024
www.cardiomyopathy.org/

Chest, Heart & Stroke, Scotland

65 North Castle Street
Edinburgh EH2 3LT
Tel: 0131 225 6963; Fax: 0131 220 6313
www.chss.org.uk/

Coronary Prevention Group – HealthNet

www.healthnet.org.uk/

Diabetes UK

10 Queen Anne Street, London W1G 9LH
Tel: 020 7323 1531; Fax: 020 7637 3644
www.diabetes.org.uk

Family Heart Association

7 North Road
Maidenhead
Berkshire SL6 1PE
Tel: 01628 628 638; Fax: 01628 628 698
www.familyheart.org

Heartlink

25 Close Street
Hemsworth
Pontefract
West Yorkshire WF9 4QP
Tel: 01977 625656
www.heartlink.org.uk

National Heart Forum

Tavistock House South
Tavistock Square
London WC1H 9LG
Tel: 0207 383 7638; Fax: 0207 387 2799
www.heartforum.org.uk/

Northern Ireland Chest Heart and Stroke Association

21 Dublin Road
Belfast BT2 7HB
Tel: 028 9032 0184; Fax: 028 9033 3487
Advice Helpline: 084 5769 7299;
Cardiac Liaison Sister Helpline: 084 5601 1658
www.nichsa.com

Stroke Association

National Helpline: 0845 30 33 100
www.stroke.org.uk/

General Practitioner

Name:
Address:
Tel:

Heart Failure Nurse

Name:
Address:
Tel:

Hospital Specialist

Name:
Address:
Tel:

Index

Abdomen, swelling, 18, 50
ACE inhibitors, 28, 29, 31
Age, 12
Air travel, 49
Alcohol, 15, 44–45
Amiloride, 29, 30
Amitriptyline, 48
Angina, 12, 14, 16, 24, 50
  exercise and, 45–46
  treatment, 32, 34–35, 48
Angioplasty, 34, 35
Angiotensin II receptor antagonists, 29, 31
Ankles, swollen, 12, 18, 30, 50
Antibiotics, 47
Anticoagulant treatment, 36–37
Antidepressant drugs, 48
Aorta, 7
Appetite, poor, 18
Arteries, 7
  see also Coronary arteries
Asthma, 48
Atherosclerosis, 14
Atrial fibrillation, 15, 32–33
Atrium, 6, 7, 8
Attitudes, of patient, 42–43, 50

Balloon angioplasty, 34, 35
Bendrofluazide, 29, 30
Beta-blockers, 28, 29, 31–32
  dosage, 32
Biopsy, 23
Bisoprolol (Cardicor), 29
Blood circulation, 6–8
  fluid retention and, 13
Blood clots, 14, 36–37
Blood pressure (high)
  see Hypertension
Blood samples, 19
Blood volume, increased, 13
Breast enlargement, 29
Breathing problems, 13, 18, 19, 50

Breathlessness, 13, 18, 19, 22–23, 30, 50
  classification of severity, 24, 25
Bronchitis, 19, 23
Bumetanide, 29, 30
Bypass surgery, 34, 35–36

Caffeine, 43
Candesartan (Amias), 29, 31
Captopril (Capoten), 29, 31
Cardiac catheterisation, 23
Cardiac glycosides, 29, 32–33
Cardiomyopathy, 15
Carvedilol (Eucardic), 29, 31, 32
Catheterisation, cardiac, 23
Chagas' disease, 15
Chest
  infections, 46–47
  pain see Angina
  X-ray, 21
Cholesterol, 14, 24
Cigarette smoking, 46
Cilazapril (Vascace), 29
Circulation see Blood circulation
Clomipramine, 48
Cold hands and feet, 32
Confusion, digoxin and, 33
Congenital heart defects, 15
Constipation, 18
Coronary arteries, 14, 23
  surgical treatment, 34–36
Coronary heart disease, 12, 13–14, 15, 24
  surgery and, 34–35
Corticosteroids, 48
Cough (dry), 18, 29, 31
Coxsackie virus, 15

Deep vein thrombosis (DVT), 49
Defibrillator, implantable, 39
Dental treatment, 47
Depression, 42

Diabetes, 12, 15, 23, 29
Diagnosis, 18–25
  classification of severity, 24–25
  confirmation, 19–23
  other illnesses and, 23–24
  symptoms, 18–19
Diarrhoea, 33
Diastole, 8
Diet, 43, 44, 45, 49
Digoxin (Lanoxin), 29, 32–33
Dilated cardiomyopathy, 15
Diltiazem, 48
Diuretics, 28, 29, 30, 43, 49
Dizziness, 18
Dothiepin, 48
Drugs
  importance, 33, 47–49, 50
  missed dose, 47
  other medications and, 28, 33, 36–37, 47, 48–49
  side-effects, 19, 28, 29, 30, 31, 32, 33, 50
  stopping medication and, 47, 48
  stopping, 33, 47
  see also specific drugs

Echocardiogram, 21, 22
Electrocardiogram (ECG), 20
Emphysema, 23
Enalapril (Innovace), 29, 31
Eprosartan (Teveten), 29, 31
Ethnic factors, 12
Exercise testing, 22
  see also Physical activity

Fatigue, 18, 25, 29, 32
Flecainide, 48
Fluid retention
  development of, 13
  in diagnosis, 18, 19
  diet and, 43, 44
  drug treatment, 29, 30
  in lungs, 13, 21, 30
Flu, immunisation, 46–47

Index

Fosinopril (Staril), 29, 31
Frusemide, 29, 30

Genetic factors, 15
Groin, swelling, 18
Gynaecomastia, 29

Hallucinations, 33
Heart attack, 12, 14, 16, 20
Heart beat, 8–9, 12
   treatment of disorders, 31, 32, 39
Heart failure, 2–3
   body's coping measures, 12–13
   causes, 13–16
   classification, 24–25
   development, 13–14
   diagnosis *see* Diagnosis
   effects on activities, 2
   incidence, 2, 12
   prevention, 16
   risk factors, 12, 15
   severity, 16, 18, 24–25
   treatment *see* Treatment
   worsening, 50
Heart failure nurse, 42–43, 50
Heart murmur, 9
Heart muscle, 13, 14
   biopsy, 23
   damaged, 9, 12–13, 14, 15
   in diagnosis, 19, 20, 21, 23
Heart (normal), 6–9
   blood circulation and, 6–8
   structure, 6, 7
   valves *see* Valves
Heart rate, 13
   drug treatment and, 32–33
   monitoring, 24
Heart rhythm
   disorders, 15, 32–33
   monitoring, 24
   testing, 20
   treatment of disorders, 39, 48
Heart sounds, 9

Heart transplantation, 34, 37–39
   suitability for, 37–38
Hereditary factors, 15
HIV infection, 15
Holidays/travel, 30, 33, 49
Holter recording, 24
Hydrochlorofluazide, 29, 30
Hyperkalaemia, 29
Hyperlipidaemia, 24
Hypertension, 14, 15, 16, 23
   drug treatment and, 30, 31, 32, 48
Hypertrophic cardiomyopathy, 15
Hypertrophy, left ventricle, 13
Hypokalaemia, 29, 30
Hyponatraemia, 29

Ibuprofen (Nurofen), 48
Imipramine, 48
Immunisation, 46–47
Impotence, 32, 49
Infections, avoidance, 46–47
Information sources, 52–54
Irbesartan (Aprovel), 29, 31

Kidneys, 13
   effects of drugs, 30, 31, 49

Left ventricular dysfunction, 13
Legs, swollen, 13, 18, 19, 30, 50
Life expectancy (increased), 30, 31, 32
Lifestyle, effects of, 16, 43–49, 50
Light-headedness, 29
Lisinopril (Zestril), 29, 31
Lithium, 48
Lofepramine, 48
Loop diuretics, 29, 30
Losartan (Cozaar), 29, 31
Lungs
   blood circulation and, 7, 8

disorders, and beta-blockers, 32
fluid retention, 13, 21, 30
function tests, 22–23

Medicines *see* Drugs; *specific drugs*
Men, 12, 29
Metoprolol (Betaloc), 29

Natriuretic peptide, 19
Nausea, 29, 33
New York Heart Association rating scale, 24, 25
Nicotine replacement therapy, 46
Nifedipine, 48
Non-steroidal anti-inflammatory drugs, 48–49
Nortriptyline, 48
Nurse (heart failure), 42–43, 50

Obesity, 15
Oedema *see* Swelling
Oxygen supply, 6, 7–8, 12–13, 14

Pacemaker
   artificial, 39
   natural, 8
Painkillers, 48
Palpitations, 25
Patient support groups, 42, 52–54
Perindopril (Coversyl), 29, 31
Physical activity
   heart beat and, 8
   recommendations, 45–46
   symptoms and, 18, 19, 25
Pill box, 33
Pneumococcal pneumonia, 47
Potassium-sparing diuretics, 29, 30
Prednisolone, 48

Pregnancy, 15
Pulmonary artery/veins, 7

Quality of life, 42
Quinapril (Accupro), 29, 31
Quinidine, 48

Ramipril (Tritace), 29, 31
Rash, 29
Rehabilitation after surgery, 36, 39
Revascularisation, coronary, 34–36
Rheumatic fever, 15
Rhythm *see* Heart rhythm

Salt
  in diet, 30, 43, 45
  failing heart and, 13
Sexual activity, 32, 49
Smoking, 46
Social support, 42
Sodium *see* Salt
Spironolactone (Aldactone), 29, 30
Stress test, 22
Support
  patient groups, 42, 52–54
  social, 42
Surgery, 33–39
  indications for, 34
  open heart, 34, 35, 36
Swelling
  abdomen, 18, 50
  feet and legs, 13, 18, 19, 30, 50
Symptoms, 2
  in classification of heart failure, 24–25
  in diagnosis, 18–19
  severity of heart failure and, 16
  worsening of, 50
Systole, 8

Telmisartan (Micardis), 29, 31

Thiazide diuretics, 29, 30
Thyroid gland, overactive, 15
Tiredness, 18, 25, 29, 32
Torasemide, 29, 30
Trandolapril (Gopten), 29
Treadmill test, 22
Treatment, 28–39
  drugs, 28–33
    ACE inhibitors, 29, 31
    angiotensin II receptor antagonists, 29, 31
    beta-blockers, 29, 31–32
    cardiac glycosides, 32–33
    diuretics, 29, 30
    importance of, 33, 47–49, 50
  effects on everyday life, 42–50
    alcohol, 15, 44–45
    diet and healthy eating, 43, 44, 45, 49
    holidays/travel and, 30, 33, 49
    importance of medicines, 47–49, 50
    infections, 46–47
    physical activity, 45–46
    sexual activity, 32, 49
    smoking, 46
    weight monitoring, 43–44, 50
  for heart rhythm disorders, 39
  surgery, 33–39
    indications for, 34
    revascularisation, 34–36
    transplantation, 37–39
    valve surgery, 36–37
Triamterene, 29

Valsartan (Diovan), 29, 31
Valves, 6
  abnormalities, 15
  damaged, 9, 14
  in diagnosis, 21, 23
  diseased, 14, 36
  surgery, 34, 36–37
Veins, 7
Ventricle, 6, 7, 8
  left, enlarged, 13, 19, 31
Verapamil, 48
Viral infections, 15
Vomiting, 29, 33

Warfarin, 36–37
Water tablets *see* Diuretics
Weakness, 18
Weight
  obesity, 15
  rapid gain, 13, 44, 50
  recording/monitoring, 30, 43–44, 50
  reduction, 16
Wheezing, 18, 29
Women, 12, 19

X-rays, 21, 23